# The Flowering of an Idea

# The Flowering of an Idea

A PLAY

PRESENTING THE ORIGIN AND EARLY DEVELOPMENT OF

THE JOHNS HOPKINS HOSPITAL

By ALAN M. CHESNEY

THE JOHNS HOPKINS UNIVERSITY PRESS
BALTIMORE

Printed in the United States of America on acid-free paper
2 4 6 8 9 7 5 3 1

The Johns Hopkins University Press
2715 North Charles Street
Baltimore, Maryland 21218-4363
www.press.jhu.edu

Library of Congress Control Number: 2009939970

ISBN 13: 978-0-8018-9432-9
ISBN 10: 0-8018-9432-8

TO

C. C. C.,

WHO PAINTED THE SCENERY FOR THIS PLAY
AND HELPED IN SO MANY OTHER WAYS,
THIS BOOK IS FONDLY DEDICATED

The reprinting of *The Flowering of an Idea,*
first published in 1939,
is sponsored by the Johns Hopkins University Press
Advisory Board in honor of Richard Ekman,
with grateful acknowledgment of his service.

# Preface

This play was written for the celebration of the fiftieth anniversary of the opening of The Johns Hopkins Hospital. It was presented in the auditorium of the Eastern High School, Baltimore, on the evening of Thursday, May 4th, 1939, by a group of players assembled and directed by Dr. N. Bryllion Fagin, Director of The Johns Hopkins Playshop.

The author's purpose in writing the play was to present some of the early events in connection with The Johns Hopkins Hospital which had an important bearing upon the subsequent development of that institution. The period covered is that which intervened between the time when Mr. Hopkins is supposed to have made up his mind how he would dispose of his fortune, a date which is uncertain but must have been earlier than 1867, and the date of the formal opening of the Hospital.

Much of the biographical material concerning Johns Hopkins which is presented in the first scene has been taken from Mrs. Helen Hopkins Thom's biography of her great uncle entitled "Johns Hopkins, a Silhouette." The author is also indebted to Dr. Charles R. Austrian, a Trustee of the Peabody Institute, for material relating to George Peabody, and to Mr. Howard A. Flynn, Governor of Sailor's Snug Harbor, for information concerning that institution. Official records of the Hospital were followed closely in the preparation of the second, third and fourth scenes. The addresses and the prayer which were given at the opening exercises of the Hospital in 1889 were considerably shortened in preparing the fourth scene as it appears in this volume. As actually presented they were curtailed even further in order to bring the last scene within the proper time limits.

# THE FLOWERING OF AN IDEA

*A Play Presenting the Origin and Early Development of The Johns Hopkins Hospital*

# *Characters*

(In the order of their first appearance)

JOHNS HOPKINS, a banker.

GEORGE PEABODY, a banker residing in London.

JAMES, a servant.

*FRANCIS T. KING, a merchant and President of the Board of Trustees of the Johns Hopkins Hospital.

*JOHN W. GARRETT, President of the Baltimore and Ohio Railroad Company.

*FRANCIS WHITE, a merchant.

*GALLOWAY CHESTON, a merchant and President of the Board of Trustees of the Johns Hopkins University.

*GEORGE W. DOBBIN, Justice of the Supreme Bench of Baltimore.

*LEWIS N. HOPKINS, a merchant, nephew of Johns Hopkins and Secretary of the Board of Trustees of the Johns Hopkins Hospital.

*THOMAS M. SMITH, a merchant.

*WILLIAM HOPKINS, a retired merchant and cousin of Johns Hopkins.

*RICHARD M. JANNEY, a retired miller, brother-in-law of Johns Hopkins.

*CHARLES J. M. GWINN, an attorney.

*Dr. ALAN P. SMITH, a physician.

*JOSEPH MERREFIELD, a merchant and later Treasurer of the Johns Hopkins Hospital.

*George W. Corner, a merchant.

*Joseph P. Elliott, a merchant.

Dr. John S. Billings, Lt. Colonel, Medical Corps, U. S. A., and Adviser to the Board of Trustees of the Johns Hopkins Hospital.

Daniel C. Gilman, President of the Johns Hopkins University and Director of the Johns Hopkins Hospital.

Rev. Joseph T. Smith, D. D., a clergyman.

Hon. Elihu E. Jackson, Governor of Maryland.

Hon. Robert C. Davidson, Mayor of Baltimore.

Dr. John Moore, Surgeon General of the United States Army.

Dr. John B. Browne, Surgeon General of the United States Navy.

Dr. John B. Hamilton, Surgeon General of the United States Public Health Service.

Mrs. Margaret Hopkins White, sister of Johns Hopkins.

Mrs. Elizbeth Schofield Hopkins, sister-in-law of Johns Hopkins.

*James Carey, a merchant.

*George William Brown, Justice of the Supreme Bench of Baltimore.

*C. Morton Stewart, a merchant.

*William T. Dixon, a merchant.

*Trustee of the Johns Hopkins Hospital.

# SCENE I.

An Imaginary Conversation in which an Idea is Born.

*Time:*—An evening in June, 1866.

*Place:*—"Clifton," the country estate of Mr. Johns Hopkins in Baltimore County.

*Characters:*—Mr. Johns Hopkins, a merchant and banker of Baltimore, 71 years of age, a Quaker and a bachelor. He is a lean man, his hair is dark and he is obviously not well-groomed. He wears a black stock.

Mr. George Peabody, a banker, formerly of Baltimore and now of London, 71 years of age, well-dressed and rather the antithesis of Mr. Hopkins. His clothes are distinctly English in their cut.

James, a colored servant.

*Scene:*—The verandah of Mr. Hopkins' house. It is a warm evening in June and as the curtain rises the two men come out of the house and look toward the city the lights of which can be seen twinkling in the distance.

## SCENE I.

*Mr. Hopkins*: I thought it would be pleasanter if we had our coffee out here. It's too good an evening to stay in-doors. Won't you have a seat? (*Indicates a chair.*)

*Mr. Peabody:* (*seating himself*) Thank you. What a splendid location you have here, Mr. Hopkins.

*Mr. Hopkins:* (*also sitting down*) I am very fond of it. I like the view you get of the city from here. And I like to see how the city is growing—each year when I move out here in the spring I think I see a difference. The houses always seem to be getting nearer and nearer, and I guess they are, too. I suppose you notice a great change in Baltimore from what it was when you left to go to London, don't you? Let me see, how long ago was that?

(*James passes the coffee.*)

*Mr. Peabody:* Just about thirty years ago—1837 it was.

*Mr. Hopkins:* As long ago as that? My, my, how time flies! Why it seems as if it were only yesterday that you were down there on German Street, selling dry goods, and I was selling groceries on Lombard Street. Lots of things have happened to the town since those days, Mr. Peabody. It's not the same place it used to be, especially since the War.

*Mr. Peabody:* I suppose not, but I have a great fondness for the place, even if I wasn't born here, and even though I have moved away. I shall never forget that it was Baltimore that gave me my start, right after the War of 1812.

(*The servant brings cigars and brandy. Mr. Hopkins takes brandy only; Mr. Peabody takes both.*)

*Mr. Peabody:* (*holding up his cigar*) You don't mind, Mr. Hopkins?

*Mr. Hopkins:* Not at all, sir, not at all. Please smoke, by all means. I guess you know I'm a Quaker and Quakers are not supposed to smoke, but I always keep a supply of cigars on hand for my guests. You will excuse me if I don't keep you company?

*Mr. Peabody:* Certainly. (*then with a smile*) I gather that the Society of Friends does not object to the use of the grape, Mr. Hopkins?

*Mr. Hopkins:* Er no, that is, not if it is taken under the doctor's orders. They don't want you to take it for pleasure and they don't want you to sell it. I ought to know. For a while I used to sell whiskey in my business, along with other things. I bought it in barrels and bottled it and labeled it "Hopkins' Best." There's a good profit in handling it that way. But I got called down by the meeting and so I quit selling it. I take a little brandy every night—my doctor says I need it at my age—says it helps my circulation. I don't know if it does. I tell my lawyer that and he just smiles and says it's another example of the wish being father to the thought.

*Mr. Peabody:* By the way, Mr. Hopkins, who is your lawyer now?

*Mr. Hopkins:* Charley Gwinn. Charles J. M. Gwinn is his full name. He's a smart young lawyer, too. I say young, he's just in his prime, I should think, his early forties. You may remember his father—he was a merchant, like ourselves.

*Mr. Peabody:* Gwinn—let me see. Oh yes, I recollect now. He imported things from the West Indies, didn't he?

*Mr. Hopkins:* Yes, that's the man. Well, his son Charley went to Princeton and did very well there, I understand. Then he read law in Latrobe's office and married Reverdy Johnson's daughter.

*Mr. Peabody:* Latrobe, did you say?

*Mr. Hopkins:* Yes. John Latrobe. He's counsel for the

B. and O. Gwinn's a splendid man and I have found that he gives very sound advice. I have him draw up all my legal papers, and I intend to name him one of my executors when I make my will.

*Mr. Peabody:* You haven't made your will yet, Mr. Hopkins?

*Mr. Hopkins:* No, Mr. Peabody, and that's just why I asked you to come here tonight. I want your advice, sir.

*Mr. Peabody:* My advice?

*Mr. Hopkins:* Yes sir, I want your advice. You see, I am getting on in years, I've accumulated a substantial fortune, I have no wife or children to leave it to, and I haven't made up my mind yet what is the best thing to do with my money. I have always looked on my wealth as a gift for which I am to be held accountable and I have always felt that it was given to me for a purpose. I don't know what that purpose is but I think that before I die I will be given to see, as we Quakers say, how I shall dispose of my estate. I regard this wealth as my stewardship.

I understand, Mr. Peabody, that you have accumulated substantial means and have made some arrangement to dispose of your fortune. I have no wish to pry into your personal concerns, sir, but if you would feel free to tell me something of what you propose to do or what you already have done, perhaps, I would be very grateful to you. I hope you will understand that I am not asking out of idle curiosity. I have a real reason for doing so. It has always been my habit to seek the best advice I could get when I was in doubt, and that's why I am asking you for yours.

*Mr. Peabody:* I feel greatly flattered, Mr. Hopkins, and I don't mind telling you in the least what I want to do and what I have already done, in fact. But before I do, let me tell you a story, if you don't object, because I think the story will give you a better idea of what I have had in mind than if I tried to give you my reasons for doing what I have.

*Mr. Hopkins:* By all means, let's have the story.

*Mr. Peabody:* Have you ever heard of a place called "Sailor's Snug Harbor"?

*Mr. Hopkins:* "Sailor's Snug Harbor"? No sir, I have never heard of it. What sort of a place is it?

*Mr. Peabody:* It's a home for old sailors, located on Staten Island, in New York Harbor. I don't suppose that you ever heard how it got started, either?

*Mr. Hopkins:* No sir, I know nothing about it. Won't you tell me?

*Mr. Peabody:* Gladly. The story concerns no less a person than Alexander Hamilton. It seems that toward the end of the last century there was a man living in New York who went by the name of Robert Randall. This man Randall inherited from his father a farm of about twenty acres located on the lower part of Manhattan Island, on what is now Fifth Avenue. It extended from about Sixth Street to Tenth Street, and East as far as what is now Fourth Avenue.

*Mr. Hopkins:* That land would be worth a lot of money now.

*Mr. Peabody:* I should say it is, and it will probably be worth a lot more in the years to come. Well, this man Randall—he was called Captain Randall—went to see Alexander Hamilton to get him to draw his will. That was along about 1800. The captain explained to Hamilton how he wished to leave his money and after Hamilton had made a note of the bequests Randall said, "I am thinking how I can dispose of the remainder of my property most wisely. What think you, General?" Whereupon Hamilton said to him:

"How did you accumulate the fortune you possess?"

"It was made for me by my father, and at his death I became his sole heir."

"How did he acquire it?" asked Hamilton.

"By honest privateering," answered Randall.

Hamilton thought a minute and then said, "Your property came from the sea. Why not give it back to the sea?"

"What do you mean?" asked Randall.

"Take your property," said Hamilton, "and found a home for the men of the sea, the old sailors, the men who helped to sail your father's privateers and all the other ships that have brought wealth to this country of ours. They helped to provide for you, now you can help to provide for them."

Randall was delighted with the idea and left practically his entire estate, which consisted mostly of the farm, for the establishment and maintenance of a home for decrepit and worn-out sailors, and he called it "Sailor's Snug Harbor." After he died some of his heirs tried to break his will,—one of the most prominent of the contestants was a bishop from Nova Scotia, so I've heard,—and the battle for the estate went on in the courts for nearly thirty years, but in the end the will was sustained and to-day "Sailor's Snug Harbor" is a very flourishing institution. I understand that the revenue from that land in rents is now so large that the institution has more money than it actually needs. I shouldn't be surprised if the income kept on getting bigger as New York grows.

*Mr. Hopkins:* That's a very interesting story.

*Mr. Peabody:* I think it is. I always liked Hamilton's idea of giving back your money to the place where your money came from, and that is why I have given some of mine to Baltimore and intend to give some more before I die.

*Mr. Hopkins:* That's a splendid sentiment, Mr. Peabody. Would you mind telling me just what you propose to do with your fortune?

*Mr. Peabody:* Not in the least. There's no secret about it. As a matter of fact, the preliminary steps were taken several years ago, before the War, and the necessary papers have already been drawn up, but the War naturally prevented my plans being carried out. I hope my Trustees will be able to start this coming autumn.

As I told you, I left Baltimore in 1837, to make my home in London, for business reasons, but I have always had a fondness for this city and I wanted to do something for the people who live here, because I feel that I owe my prosperity in large measure to Baltimore. It was here that I was able to get my start in business and make enough money to get ahead and go into banking.

Well, in 1857 I picked out twenty-five trustees from friends of mine in whom I have confidence, and I gave them a letter of instructions and three hundred thousand dollars to start with, and a promise of more to come. I told them that I wanted to establish and endow an Institute in Baltimore to improve the culture of the inhabitants of the city and the state, and to help spread a taste for the fine arts. I told them specifically that I wanted to provide an extensive library, not the ordinary kind of lending library but one for reference and study, where students could get hold of books that wouldn't be found in the usual library. Then I would like to see every year lectures on science, art, and literature, and I would like to provide cash prizes and medals to be given every year to the boys and girls graduating from the high schools of Baltimore with the best records. I am in hopes that these prizes may encourage the young people of the city to study harder. I also instructed my Trustees to provide an Academy of Music, to cultivate and spread a taste for music, which has always been to me the most refining of all the arts. I told them I wanted the Institute to have a Gallery of Art, supplied as far as possible with the works of the best masters, where artists could study and make copies of the paintings if they wanted to, and I hope that it will be possible to have an annual exhibition in that gallery.

In general, Mr. Hopkins, the idea I had in mind was to improve the opportunities in Baltimore for culture. I would like to have founded a college or a university but I did not have money enough for that. After all, there is such a thing as spreading one's gifts too thin, I suppose. I hope to complete the endowment by autumn of this year, and in fact that's why I am in this country now. I hope it will be possible to open the Institute soon, for it has already been delayed a long time, largely on account of the War and for other reasons that I shall not go into now.

*Mr. Hopkins:* That's a splendid program, Mr. Peabody, and I'm very much obliged to you for telling me about it. What a fine thing to do for the city of Baltimore! The citizens of this community will owe an everlasting debt of gratitude to you, sir.

*Mr. Peabody:* Oh, I don't care about that. I got my start here—the people of Baltimore helped to make my fortune for me and I feel that I am only paying back something that I owe them. By the way, Mr. Hopkins, were you born in Baltimore?

*Mr. Hopkins:* No, sir. I was born down in Anne Arundel County, near South River. My father owned a large tobacco plantation there, about 500 acres, and enough slaves to take care of the land. We had a very good living from it until my father freed his slaves.

*Mr. Peabody:* When did he do that?

*Mr. Hopkins:* Oh, about 1807, I think. I was only twelve years old at the time.

*Mr. Peabody:* That was a long time before the War, wasn't it? What made him do it, anyway?

*Mr. Hopkins:* The Meeting of the Society of Friends—we were Quakers, you know,—voted that everyone must free his slaves or be dropped from the Meeting. My father was a loyal Quaker. He accepted the decision of his church—and freed his slaves. That is all there was to it.

*Mr. Peabody:* It must have been rather hard on the family.

*Mr. Hopkins:* Yes, it was, especially on my mother. We were a large family, and she had to do many things for us that the slaves used to do. She made all of our clothes for us, even to spinning the thread. But I often think that in the end it was a good thing for all of us and certainly it was for me, because otherwise I might not have been forced to come to Baltimore and go in business, if my father had kept his slaves.

*Mr. Peabody:* And you never married?

*Mr. Hopkins:* No, sir. I thought of doing so once—I wanted to marry my cousin, Elisabeth Hopkins, but her father, my father's brother, wouldn't allow us to wed. The Society of Friends did not look with favor on the marriage of first cousins, and I could never persuade Uncle Gerard to change his mind. At any rate, his refusal made me go in business for myself, and it was in business and later in banking that I made my money, in very much the same way that you did, yourself, sir. And now I wish to arrange for the disposal of my fortune after I'm gone. What would you suggest that I do with it? You mentioned that you didn't have enough to start a college or a university.

*Mr. Peabody:* No, I know I haven't enough to do that. If you have enough to do it, I would think it would be a fine way to use your wealth. I can't think of a better place in which to start a college or a university than Baltimore. Look at all the young men in the South who will be wanting to go back to studying, now that the War is over. They have been so hard hit in the South that their own schools and colleges will have a hard job of it getting back on their feet.

*Mr. Hopkins:* That's certainly true. And I owe something to the South for I've done a lot of business there in my time, especially in Virginia and North Carolina.

*Mr. Peabody:* Of course, there are other things you might do with your money. You might found a hospital.

*Mr. Hopkins:* I had thought of that, myself. Dr. Parrish, of Philadelphia, also made that suggestion.

*Mr. Peabody:* Aren't there always plenty of sick people in Baltimore? Or is it a much healthier place than it used to be when I lived here?

*Mr. Hopkins:* I doubt if it is much healthier than it was then. It seems as if almost every day I hear of one of my friends getting typhoid fever or malaria, and some of them die, too. I wonder if the doctors will ever learn how to get rid of those diseases for us.

*Mr. Peabody:* I fancy they will. Just look at what vaccination has done to wipe out smallpox. But it will take a lot of hard work and hard study. I have great faith in the future, however. I think our educational institutions and our doctors will do a lot to make life happier for the next generation and the generations after that. I wouldn't be surprised if some day typhoid fever and malaria would be almost as unheard of in Baltimore as smallpox is now. But you've got to give the doctors a chance to work at them, Mr. Hopkins. (looks at his watch and rises) I'm afraid I must be going, and I'm afraid I've talked too much already. I hope I haven't tired you. It has been a delightful evening.

*Mr. Hopkins:* It has been a delightful evening for me, Mr. Peabody, and I am greatly obliged to you for coming and for your very helpful advice. You have given me a lot to think about. One moment, while I call the carriage. (*summons the servant, who enters*) James, will you call the carriage for Mr. Peabody?

*James:* Yas, sir, it's all ready at the stable, sir.

*Mr. Hopkins:* And bring Mr. Peabody's things, please. (*then, as the servant leaves, he turns to Mr. Peabody*) Are you staying in Baltimore for some time?

*Mr. Peabody:* Only for a few days to settle some details with my Trustees. I am not going back to England until the fall, but I shall be going North for the summer. I was born in Massachusetts, and I'll be going there for the summer months.

(*James appears with Mr. Peabody's hat, walking stick and shawl. He hands the hat and stick to Mr. Peabody and then drapes the shawl over his shoulders.*)

(*to James*) Thank you.
(*to Mr. Hopkins*) I find this comfortable when I am driving at night.

*Mr. Hopkins:* Yes, by all means keep yourself warm. It is surprising how chilly you can get these summer evenings when you ride behind fast-stepping horses. You'll find that's a lively pair that is taking you into town tonight.

*Mr. Peabody:* Well, good night, sir, and thank you once more for a very pleasant evening. (*shakes hands with Mr. Hopkins*)

*Mr. Hopkins:* Good night, and thank you for coming. I hope you have a pleasant voyage back to England in the autumn.

*Mr. Peabody:* Thank you. Good night. (*Mr. Peabody departs*)

(*Mr. Hopkins escorts him to the steps, then comes*

*back, stands for a moment looking at the city, then seats himself and talks aloud to himself.*)

*Mr. Hopkins:* A university or a hospital?—Why shouldn't I do both? That's an idea! There ought to be enough money for the two. Let me see. The University could be located here at Clifton,—the Hospital would have to be located in town, nearer where the sick folks are. Perhaps there could be a broad avenue connecting the two that would beautify the city. The University would have to have a medical school, of course, but that oughtn't to be located here at Clifton. That would have to be where the Hospital is, because the Hospital would be absolutely necessary to the Medical School, and the Medical School ought to help the work of the Hospital, I should think. I don't know why not. The thing to do is to make sure that the Medical School and the Hospital are so tied up to one another that there can never be any question of their not working together. That oughtn't to be hard to fix. I must make a note of it at once and get Gwinn to draw up the necessary papers. James!

(*James appears in the doorway.*)

*James:* Yas, sir.

*Mr. Hopkins:* Bring me a pen and ink and some paper,

will you? (*takes out his spectacles and adjusts them in place*)

*James:* Yas, sir. (*shuffles out and returns in a moment with a pen, ink bottle, pad and lamp. Arranges these on a small table*)

*Mr. Hopkins:* Thanks. That'll be all. (*James leaves*) (*Mr. Hopkins writes slowly, pronouncing each word that he writes*) Hospital to form part of Medical School of University provided for by my will.

CURTAIN.

## SCENE II.

A Special Meeting of the Board of Trustees of the Hospital.

*Time:*—March 11, 1873.

*Place:*—An office in Baltimore.

*Characters:*—Mr. Francis T. King, President of the Board, Messrs. John W. Garrett, Francis White, Galloway Cheston, (Judge) George W. Dobbin, Lewis N. Hopkins, Thomas M. Smith, William Hopkins, Richard M. Janney, Charles J. M. Gwinn, (Dr.) Alan P. Smith and Joseph Merrefield, all Trustees of the Hospital. As the curtain rises the Trustees are discovered seated around a table chatting with one another.

## SCENE II.

M*r. King:* Will the meeting please come to order? As this is a special meeting of the Board, we will dispense with the reading of the minutes of the previous meeting, unless some member wishes to have them read. (*Pauses. No wish is expressed. He continues.*) I do not hear any one speak so we shall proceed. I have called this special meeting in order that the Board may hear a communication from the founder of the institution, who is also our esteemed friend. Before I ask the Secretary to read the communication I would inform you, officially, what I daresay all of you know, that Mr. Hopkins has purchased the tract of land in East Baltimore which is now occupied by the buildings of the old Maryland Hospital for the Insane. He purchased it with the understanding that the streets which have been laid through it would be permanently closed. The necessary ordinances have been passed by the City Council, I am glad to say, and they have been ratified by the State Legislature, so that that question is settled. The deed transferring the property to this Board has been executed and recorded, and is now in our possession. The communication which I shall now ask the Secretary to read, is, I understand, a letter of instructions to this Board.

Mr. Secretary, will you be good enough to read Mr. Hopkins' letter?

Mr. Lewis Hopkins (*reads*):

"Baltimore, March 10th, 1873.

"To Francis T. King, President: and John W. Garrett, Hon. Geo. W. Dobbin, Galloway Cheston, Thomas M. Smith, Wm. Hopkins, Richard M. Janney, Joseph Merrefield, Francis White, Lewis N. Hopkins, Alan P. Smith, and Charles J. M. Gwinn, Trustees of 'The Johns Hopkins Hospital':

"Gentlemen:

"I have given you in your capacity of Trustees, thirteen acres of land, situated in the city of Baltimore, and bounded by Wolfe, Monument, Broadway and Jefferson streets, upon which I desire you to erect a hospital. It will be necessary to devote the present year to the grading of its surface, to its proper drainage, to the laying out of the grounds, and the most careful and deliberate choice of a plan for the erection and arrangement of the new hospital buildings. It is my wish that the plan thus chosen shall be one which will permit symmetrical additions to the buildings which will be first constructed, in order that you may ultimately be able to receive four hundred patients, and that it shall provide for an hospital which shall in construction and arrangement compare favorably with any other institution of like character in this country or in Europe. It will therefore be your duty to obtain the advice and assistance of those at home or abroad who have achieved the greatest success in the construction and management of hospitals. I cannot press this injunction too strongly upon you, because the usefulness of this charity will greatly depend upon the plan which you may adopt for the construction and arrangement of the buildings. It is my desire that you should complete this portion of your labor during the current year, and be in readiness to commence the building of the hospital in the spring of 1874.

"It will be your duty hereafter to provide for the erection upon other ground, of suitable buildings for the reception, maintenance and education of orphan colored children. I direct you to provide accommodation for three or four hundred children of this class; and you are also authorized to receive into this asylum, at your discretion, as belonging to such class, colored children who have lost one parent only, and in exceptional cases to receive colored children who are not orphans, but may be in such circumstances as to require the aid of charity. I desire that you shall apply the yearly sum of twenty thousand dollars, or so much thereof as may be necessary, of the revenue of the property which you will hereafter receive, to the maintenance of the Orphans' Home intended for such children.

"In order to enable you to carry my wishes into full effect, I will now, and in each succeeding year during my life until the hospital buildings are fully completed and in readiness to receive patients, place at your disposal the sum of one hundred thousand dollars. In addition to the gift already made to you of the thirteen acres of land in the city of Baltimore upon which the hospital will be built, I have dedicated to its support and the payment of the annual sum provided to be paid for the support of the Orphans' Home, property which you may safely estimate as worth to-day two million of dollars, and from which your corporation will certainly receive a yearly revenue of one hundred and twenty thousand dollars, and which time and your diligent care will make more largely productive. If the Hospital and Orphans' Home are not built at my death, it will be your duty to apply the income arising from this property to their completion. When they are built, the income from the property will suffice for the maintenance. The indigent sick of this city and its environs, without regard to sex, age, or color, who require surgical or medical treatment, and who can be received into the hospital without peril to the other inmates, and the poor of the city and State, of all races, who are stricken down by any casualty, shall be received into the hospital without charge, for such periods of time and under such regulations as you may prescribe. It will be your duty to make such division of the sexes and patients among the several wards of the hospital as will best promote the actual usefulness of the charity. You will also provide for the reception of a limited number of patients who are able to make compensation for the room and attention they may require. The money received from such persons will enable you to appropriate a larger sum for the relief of the sufferings of that class which I direct you to admit free of charge, and you will thus be enabled to afford to strangers, and to those of our own people who have no friends or relatives to care for them in sickness, and who are not objects of charity, the advantage of careful and skillful treatment.

"It will be your especial duty to secure for the service of the hospital, surgeons and physicians of the highest character and of the greatest skill. I desire you to establish, in connection with the hospital, a training school for female nurses. This provision will secure the services of women competent to care for the sick in the hospital wards, and will enable you to benefit the whole community by supplying it with a class of trained and experienced nurses.

"I wish the large grounds surrounding the hospital buildings to be properly enclosed by iron railings, and to be so laid out and planted with trees and flowers as to afford solace to the sick and be an ornament to the section of the city in which the grounds are located. I desire that you should, in due season, provide for a site and buildings of such description and at such distance from the city as your judgment shall approve, for the reception of convalescent patients. You will be able in this way to hasten the recovery of the sick, and to have always room in the main hospital building for other sick persons requiring immediate medical or surgical treatment. It is my special request that the influences of religion should be felt in and impressed upon the whole management of the hospital; but I desire, nevertheless, that the administration of the charity shall be undisturbed by sectarian influences, discipline, or control. In all your arrangements in relation to this hospital, you will bear constantly in mind that it is my wish and purpose that the institution should ultimately form a part of the medical school of that university for which I have made ample provision by my will. I have felt it to be my duty to bring these subjects to your particular attention, knowing that you will conform to the wishes which I definitely express. In other particulars I leave your board to the exercise of its discretion, believing that your good judgment and experience in life will enable you to make this charity a substantial benefit to the community.

"I am very respectfully your friend,

"Johns Hopkins."

*Mr. King:* It is not necessary for me to comment upon the importance of the communication which we have just heard. It conveys the wishes of the founder of this trust, and as his Trustees we are all bound to carry out his instructions in as loyal a fashion as possible. Are there any comments?

*Mr. Cheston:* Mr. President, I think that this letter from Mr. Hopkins should be printed so that each of us may have a copy of it to study carefully. I move you, sir, that 500 copies be printed for distribution to the proper parties.

*Mr. King:* Is there a second to Mr. Cheston's motion?

*Mr. Garrett:* I second it.

*Mr. King:* Is there any discussion? (*Pauses. Silence.*) If not, will all those in favor of Mr. Cheston's motion please say "aye."

(*Chorus of "ayes"*)

*Mr. King:* Those opposed will please say "No." (*Pauses*) The motion is carried. Mr. Secretary, will you please be good enough to arrange for the printing? Any further comment? (*Pauses*) If not, I will present for your consideration the proposed composition of the committees which were authorized at the last meeting of the Board. By action of the Board taken at that time, it is understood that the President of the Board will be ex-officio chairman of each of these committees. The list is as follows: (*reads from list*)

*Building Committee:* Messrs. Galloway Cheston, George W. Dobbin, John W. Garrett, Alan P. Smith and Charles J. M. Gwinn.

*Finance Committee:* Messrs. John W. Garrett, Galloway Cheston, Thomas M. Smith.

*By-Laws:* Messrs. Charles J. M. Gwinn and George W. Dobbin.

*Miscellaneous Business:* Francis White, William Hopkins and Richard M. Janney.

*Mr. Garrett:* Mr. President, I move that the list be approved as read.

*Mr. White:* I second the motion, Mr. President.

*Mr. King:* You have all heard the motion. Is there any discussion? (*Pauses a moment*) If not, will all in favor please say "aye."

(*Chorus of "ayes"*)

*Mr. King:* Those opposed will please say "No." (*Pauses. Silence.*) So ordered. Is there any further business? If not, the chair will entertain a motion to adjourn.

*Mr. Gwinn:* I move we adjourn.

*Chorus:* I second the motion. (*All rise as the curtain falls.*)

CURTAIN.

## SCENE III.

A Meeting of the Board of Trustees of
the Johns Hopkins Hospital.

*Time:*—February 20, 1877.

*Place:*—An office at 25 N. Charles Street, Baltimore, provided with a blackboard.

*Characters:*—Mr. Francis T. King, President of the Board, Messrs. John W. Garrett, Francis White, Galloway Cheston, (Judge) George W. Dobbin, Lewis N. Hopkins, Thomas M. Smith, William Hopkins, Charles J. M. Gwinn, (Dr.) Alan P. Smith, George W. Corner and Joseph P. Elliott, all Trustees of the Hospital, and Dr. John S. Billings.

As the curtain rises the Trustees are discovered seated around the table. Mr. Lewis Hopkins, the Secretary, is finishing the reading of the minutes of the previous meeting.

## SCENE III.

*Mr. Hopkins:* . . . There being no further business the meeting then adjourned.

*Mr. King:* Are there any corrections to these minutes? (*Pauses for a moment*) If not, they stand approved as read. We will now proceed to the principal business of the meeting which is to hear a report from Dr. Billings concerning the progress he has made on the plans which he has prepared for the Hospital. Dr. Billings, will you be good enough to take the floor?

*Dr. Billings:* Certainly, Mr. President.

(*Rises, goes over to the blackboard, unrolls a large scale drawing which he proceeds to hang on the blackboard.*)

Gentlemen, I have had the architect, Mr. Niernsee, draw this block plan to show the layout of the buildings as I think they should be built. They are arranged in accordance with the general principles which have already been adopted by the Building Committee. As you will see, the main entrance of the Hospital is on Broadway, through the Administration Building. On either side of it is a ward for private patients. These three buildings are connected with one another by a corridor, which also connects with the other wards.

I have planned the Hospital on the pavilion system as I consider this to be the best for all purposes. The wards are one story buildings, resting on basements about ten feet high, and the top of the corridor is on a level with the ward floors so that it will form a walk or veranda from one ward to another. Upon the south side of the grounds an open space is provided for tents, which are to be used for cases not suitable for the common or isolation wards. The number of beds which this plan will accommodate is 400.

The buildings of the Medical Department of the University will be on a square diagonally across from the northeast corner of the Hospital, and the Amphitheatre and Pathological building are placed with reference to this location. On the south is the nurses' building and on the north is the kitchen. The administration building has three floors. The first or main floor is for office and business purposes; the second for the resident medical staff; the third for the resident medical students.

As I have previously stated, it is my idea that the Medical School of the University has an opportunity to do work which is either not done at all, or is not done in the best manner elsewhere in this country. In my opinion it should train men to be original investigators, bring them face to face with the innumerable problems relating to life and death and disease, and inspire them with the desire to investigate these questions. I think that the classes should be small, not more than twenty-five each, and that the entire senior class should live in the Hospital and assume the care of patients under the supervision of the resident medical staff. I have planned the third floor of the administration building so as to accommodate these twenty-five students. (*Pauses*)

*Mr. King:* Are there any questions that any one would like to ask Dr. Billings?

*Mr. White:* Did you show these plans to any one while you were abroad last Fall, Dr. Billings?

*Dr. Billings:* Yes, Mr. White. With regard to the general plan of the Hospital, I can only say that it is approved by the majority of the experts to whom I have submitted it. I do not think we have much to learn from Europe as regards the general principles of hospital construction and management, or as regards heating and ventilation; in fact these things cannot be said as yet to be settled on any scientific basis of observed facts, and there are nearly as many opinions as persons. Surprise was freely expressed at my coming from America to Europe to learn about hospitals. The general tendency in the most recent hospitals is, however, towards one story wards, especially for surgical and medical cases, or those for which the best possible surroundings are desired, and towards separation and isolation of the several buildings. That is the arrangement of the new City Hospital in Berlin, which was planned by Professor Virchow.

*Dr. Smith:* Is there any evidence to show that one type of hospital construction gives better results in the care of patients than other types?

*Dr. Billings:* I did not find it possible to obtain positive reliable data on that point, Dr. Smith. Mortality statistics are of no use for this purpose, since the character of the patients received varies so much. Indeed, I came back more thoroughly impressed and convinced than ever, that the thing of prime importance in a hospital is minute care of, and cleanliness in, every part and person about it, and in the management and supervision which will insure this, while without it the most perfect hospital that can be built soon deteriorates and gives only second or third rate results. It is not possible to say how much healthier one story wards are, than those of two or more, or how much better results will be obtained by having the wards separated, and giving to each the greatest possible air space. The general opinion is that these one story isolation wards are the best of all, but I cannot learn what increased percentage of recoveries they will insure. After careful reflection, I advise the Trustees to adhere to the principle of the central garden, and to the one story pavilion, with the exception of the two nearest the administration building, which may be of two stories, while advantage may be taken of the space thus gained, to obtain more room on the Broadway front, and elevation for the buildings.

*Mr. King:* Is not the pavilion plan more expensive than the old convent plan?

*Dr. Billings:* Undoubtedly, and I do not underestimate the importance of that fact.

*Mr. Garrett:* Have you made any estimate of the cost of your proposed plan?

*Dr. Billings:* Yes, Mr. Garrett, I have. I estimate that if the Hospital is built on this plan, calculating for plain but good and substantial work and omitting all architectural ornament and decoration, except for the main front or memorial buildings, it will cost when furnished $1,200,000. As it is necessary, by the terms of the trust, that the expense of construction shall be met from annual income, and as the first year's income has been wisely applied to enlarging the grounds, it follows that if this plan is adopted, the Hospital cannot be ready for operations before the autumn of 1880.

*Mr. Garrett:* That means a considerable delay, does it not?

*Dr. Billings:* Yes, Mr. Garrett. In fact, I think there are just two courses open to the Trustees.

*Mr. King:* What are they?

*Dr. Billings:* The first is to accept the estimates offered as being as nearly correct as such things can be, approve the general plan and arrangement now prepared and authorize the preparation of working drawings on the basis of these estimates. The second course which may be taken by the Trustees is to decide that the buildings *must* be put up more cheaply.

*Mr. King:* Which course do you recommend?

*Dr. Billings:* Gentlemen, I have given very serious consideration to the question whether the Hospital should be built more cheaply, and on a less ambitious plan. I cannot convince myself that it should. If the Hospital, to use the words of Johns Hopkins, is to "compare favorably with any other institution of like character in this country or in Europe," if it is to furnish the best treatment and accommodations for patients, promote advance in medical science, secure, retain and improve such medical officers and nurses as are desired, and form a suitable memorial to its founder, it will cost at least one million dollars. I respectfully recommend that plans on this basis be authorized.

If this be not approved, then I recommend that *all* the buildings be built with regard to cheapness mainly, at a total cost of about $350,000, abandoning entirely the general plan of which I have been speaking.

I advise that no attempt at a compromise between these two courses be attempted, for if it is, the result will be satisfactory to nobody.

(*Several Trustees nod their heads to show their acquiescence.*)

*Mr. White:* Mr. President, has the Building Committee studied these plans?

*Mr. King:* I am glad that you asked that question, Mr. White. The Building Committee has gone over them carefully with Dr. Billings and has unanimously voted to recommend to this Board that Dr. Billings' recommendation be adopted, namely that the plans submitted by him be approved and the Hospital constructed on that basis, it being understood that the entire cost will probably exceed one million dollars.

*Mr. Gwinn:* I move that the recommendation of the Building Committee be approved.

(*Chorus of "I second the motion."*)

*Mr. King:* You have heard the motion. Is there any discussion?

*Mr. Garrett:* Mr. President.

*Mr. King:* Mr. Garrett.

*Mr. Garrett:* I concur in this motion and shall vote for it, but I wish now to express the hope that the step we are about to take will not delay too long the opening of the Hospital. I think that the time may come when we will wish to open the Hospital even if all of the wards are not completed, and I would like to have it understood that this action does not bind us not to open the Hospital for partial operation until the last brick is safely in place.

*Dr. Smith:* I fully agree with Mr. Garrett, Mr. President.

*Mr. King:* I understand your position, Mr. Garrett, and I do not consider that this action in any way binds us as to the time the Hospital shall be open for the reception of patients. Is that clear, Dr. Billings?

*Dr. Billings:* Perfectly.

*Mr. King:* Any further discussion? (*Pauses*) If not, are you ready for the question? (*Pauses*) All in favor of the motion will please say "Aye."

(*Chorus of "Ayes."*)

Those opposed, "No."

(*Silence.*)

The ayes have it. Mr. Secretary, will you please record the vote as unanimous. Gentlemen, before we adjourn, I wish to express, on behalf of the Board, our great gratitude to Dr. Billings for the careful attention he has given to this question and for the valuable help he has given us. I am sure that the step we have taken to-day is a most important one for the future of the Johns Hopkins Hospital. The meeting stands adjourned.

CURTAIN.

## SCENE IV.

The Hospital is Opened.

*Time:*—May 7, 1889, 11:00 A. M.

*Place:*—The Johns Hopkins Hospital.

*Characters:*—Mr. Francis T. King, President of the Board of Trustees, Mr. Daniel C. Gilman, President of the Johns Hopkins University, Col. Johns S. Billings, U. S. A., Rev. Joseph T. Smith, D. D., of Baltimore.

The Governor of the State, the Mayor of the City, the Surgeons General of the Army, Navy and Public Health Service, the following Trustees, Francis White, Judge George W. Dobbin, Lewis N. Hopkins, Charles J. M. Gwinn, Dr. Alan P. Smith, Joseph P. Elliott, George W. Corner, James Carey, George William Brown, C. Morton Stewart, William T. Dixon, and two ladies, the only surviving sister and sister-in-law of Johns Hopkins, are all seated on a platform facing the audience.

Beside the rostrum there is a marble bust of Johns Hopkins. The platform is decorated with flowers and two flags—American and Maryland. It is located in the rotunda of the Hospital. There is the sound of a string orchestra playing as the curtain rises. In a moment it ceases.

## SCENE IV.

M*r. King:* (*rising*) Ladies and Gentlemen: Johns Hopkins, in his letter to his Trustees, said: "It is my special request that the influence of religion should be felt in and impressed upon the whole management of the Hospital; but I desire nevertheless that the administration of charity shall be undisturbed by sectarian influence, discipline or control." It is therefore most appropriate that we should begin the opening exercises of the Hospital by reverently waiting upon God, and asking His blessing upon this work and His abiding presence within these walls, which are to be devoted to the care of the sick and suffering. I will therefore call upon the Reverend Dr. Joseph T. Smith for prayer.

(*The company on the platform stand.*)

*Rev. Smith:* (*advancing to centre of platform, prays. The company bow their heads reverently*) Most merciful and gracious God, our heavenly Father! We worship Thee, we praise Thee, we magnify Thy name as the God in whom we live and move and have our being and from whose kind hand cometh down every good gift and every perfect gift which we enjoy. In all our ways we would acknowledge Thee, for Thou art God alone. Upon all the works of our hands we would seek Thy benediction, for Thy blessing alone can prosper.

We bless Thee for all the alleviations Thou hast provided for pain and for all the remedies Thou hast provided to mitigate, where they cannot remove disease; for these healing waters compounded in Thine own hidden laboratory; for these healing plants which Thou has caused to grow in garden, and field, and forest; for these healing minerals which Thou hast stored away, with the silver and the gold in the mines, furnishing the hospital earth so abundantly with all needful supplies for its sick and impotent folk. We thank Thee for the pity Thou hast implanted in human hearts, and the skill Thou hast given to physicians to discover and administer the remedies Thou hast provided, so and ever increasingly lessening the sum of human suffering.

And now that this great company is gathered here from their wide dispersion on this day of gladness, which crowns the cares and labors of so many years, our hearts rise up to Thee in thanksgiving and praise. As we look around on this Bethesda, this house of mercy, with its many apartments so admirably constructed, so abundantly furnished with all needful appliances, we thank Thee that Thou didst put into the heart of Thy servant, who so long went in and out among us, to provide so munificently for the building of this hospital. We thank Thee for the Grace given to these, Thy servants, to whom, as he was about to go into the far country, he left his goods, to fulfil with such wisdom and fidelity their high trust.

Bless and reward abundantly, for their labor of love, Thy servants who have given so many years of care and toil to the erection of these buildings. Bless the physicians and nurses who shall from time to time be employed here with wisdom and skill and tenderness. Bless all who shall in any way be employed in the service of this hospital, and let Thy choicest benedictions rest upon the sufferers who shall be gathered here from generation to generation. Amen.

(*The company seat themselves.*)

*Mr. King:* (*rises and goes to rostrum with manuscript*) Ladies and Gentlemen: It is my pleasant duty, in behalf of the Trustees of the Johns Hopkins Hospital, to offer you a cordial welcome, and to express our high appreciation of the interest in our work which is manifested by your presence here to-day.

It cannot be a matter of small or temporary

importance that brings to this opening the chief executives of our State and our City, so many of our distinguished men in all branches of the public service, so many well-known professional men from distant cities and countries, and so many of our own most prominent and public-spirited citizens: and it gives us a renewed sense of our responsibilities and duties to find that we are to give an account of what we have done in the past and we hope to do in the future to such an audience as we see before and around us.

Johns Hopkins did not leave a hospital; what he did leave was a complicated piece of machinery in the form of various investments capable of evolving the power required to construct and maintain a hospital, for in this sense money is power. This machinery requires constant adjustment and looking after, and for this part of the work the Trustees are solely responsible.

When I tell you that these seventeen buildings have been constructed and furnished, and these fourteen and a half acres enclosed and beautified as you see them to-day, not only without taking a dollar from the principal placed in the hands of the Trustees, but with an actual increase of the endowment by judicious investments by the sum of one hundred and thirteen thousand dollars, I think it may be justly claimed that the Trustees have not failed in this part of their duty. (*Applause*)

I wish to say, on behalf of the Trustees, a few words of recognition to all who have labored to bring these plans to their conclusion; to the medical adviser (*bows to Col. Billings*), whose invaluable services have covered more than ten years; to the President of the University (*bows to President Gilman*), who has so ably aided in organizing; to the architects and builders, and to those who have had but occasional opportunities to serve us, but who have freely contributed their wisdom and experience whenever called upon, and especially to the physicians and surgeons, the managers of other hospitals, the superintendents of training schools for nurses, and to many others, at home and abroad, whose kind cooperation has been most serviceable.

As Johns Hopkins was brought up by godly parents—members of the Society of Friends,—I should have been glad if we might have heard the voice of Whittier, the Quaker poet, but in the letter which I hold in my hand (*holds up letter*) he pleads his age and illness as an excuse for his silence. He expresses his pleasure in seeing that the wise and benevolent design of the founder has been so well carried out, and his hope that the example of Johns Hopkins will not be lost upon his country.

To the words of his letter I will venture to add this verse, which he wrote for another occasion, but which is equally appropriate for this:—

"Not vainly the gift of its founder was made;
Not prayerless the stones of its corner were laid;
To Him be the glory forever!—we bear
To the Lord of the Harvest our wheat with the tare;
What we lack in our work, may He find in our will,
And winnow in mercy our good from the ill."

(*Turns and sits down. Applause. As the applause dies down he rises and again steps forward.*)

*Mr. King:* It is now my pleasure to call upon the man who planned the buildings of this Hospital and who has watched over its construction from the very beginning. A member of the Medical Corps of the United States Army with a distinguished career in the late War between the States, he has made a great name for himself as an authority on sanitation and hospital construction. He was one of the five distinguished experts on hospital construction who were invited to submit plans for the Hospital, and his essay on this subject was such as to lead the Trustees to request the Surgeon General of the Army that he be allowed to serve in the capacity of expert adviser in the planning and supervising of the construction of the Hospital. I wish to take this opportunity to express publicly our great debt of gratitude not only to this man but also to Surgeon General Barnes for his whole-hearted cooperation in this matter. It gives me great pleasure to present to you Dr. John Shaw Billings, Colonel in the Medical Corps of the United States Army. (*Applause*)

*Dr. Billings:* (*rises and comes forward with a manuscript from which he reads*) Mr. President, ladies and gentlemen: The third paragraph of the letter of instructions communicated by Johns Hopkins to the Trustees whom he had chosen to carry out his plans for a hospital in the city of Baltimore, states that "it is my wish that this plan . . . shall provide a Hospital which shall in structure and arrangement, compare favorably with any other institution of like character in this country or in Europe." What do you suppose the writer was thinking of when he penned that sentence? Had he in view any definite ideal; any mental picture of the institution which he proposed to establish; or was it merely an expression of a desire to give to his city the best thing that could be devised?

To "compare favorably with"—what does that mean? It is a peculiar phrase, which, coming from a shrewd business man and a member of the Society of Friends, signifies, I think, to excel, if possible; at all events, that is the safest interpretation. And it was not this or that hospital which was to be surpassed or equaled, but all other hospitals in this country or in Europe—Africa, Asia and Australia being put out of the question. It was a large contract.

Let us now consider the broad general principles which governed the Trustees in the adoption of the plan for the Hospital. The first hospitals were established to give shelter and food to the sick poor, especially those who gathered in cities. Gradually physicians found that they could learn much in these aggregations of suffering and that they afforded the means of teaching others; but this last use of them is only about two hundred years old. Gradually, also, it came to be known that the knowledge thus obtained in the care of the sick poor was of use in treating the diseases of the well-to-do; and finally, within the last twenty-five years or so, people are beginning to find out that when they are afflicted with certain forms of disease or injury they can be better treated in a properly appointed hospital than they can be in their own homes, no matter how costly or luxurious these may be. This Hospital, then, is to provide for the rich as well as the poor; for those who can, and ought to, pay for the help given, as well as for those who cannot.

A second cardinal principle to be observed in such a hospital as this, is that it shall do as little harm as possible. A hospital may do harm by its foul air, by spreading contagious disease among its inmates, by neglect or carelessness of its nurses or attendants; and in years gone by hospitals have, no doubt, caused nearly as much sickness as they have relieved. This is now rarely the case, and in this hospital the arrangements for ventilation, isolation, and nursing are such as to entirely do away with this danger.

The third principle to be kept in view in such a hospital as this is that it should provide the means of giving medical instruction; for the sake of the sick in the institution as well as those out of it. It is well known to those familiar with the subject that the sick in a hospital where medical instruction is given receive more constant, careful, and thoughtful attention than do those in a hospital where no such instruction is given. The clinical teacher must do his best; keen eyes will note every error in diagnosis, every failure in results of treatment. Moreover, the very act of teaching clarifies and crystallizes his own knowledge; in attempting to explain, the dark places become prominent and demand investigation; and hence it is that those cases which are lectured on receive the best treatment. I need say nothing here on the other side of the question, the value of properly trained physicians to the community and the necessity for hospital instruction in such training; Johns Hopkins understood all this and specially directed that "in all your arrangements in relation to this Hospital you will bear constantly in mind that it is my wish and purpose that the institution shall ultimately form a part of the Medical School of the University."

Another point which had to be kept in view was the direction of Mr. Hopkins that there should be established "in connection with the hospital, a training school for female nurses, not only to care for the sick in the hospital, but to benefit the whole community, by supplying it with a class of trained and experienced nurses."

It is also highly desirable that a hospital of this kind should have connected with it a well-appointed dispensary for the treatment of those who need medical aid, but not a bed in a hospital.

The last point to which I shall refer, which was

kept in view by the Trustees in deciding upon the plans, was the general appearance of the buildings and grounds.

Mr. Hopkins gave no specific directions as to the buildings, but he directed that the grounds should be properly enclosed by iron railings, and so laid out and planted as to be a solace to the sick and an ornament to the city, and it was evident that the buildings should be of the same character so far as their purpose would admit.

These, then, were the main principles—to provide for the proper care of the sick, both rich and poor, to provide for the highest class of medical education, to increase and diffuse knowledge, to provide trained nurses for both hospital and city, to provide a dispensary, and to make the buildings and grounds ornamental and attractive.

On the philanthropic, social and religious aspects of this great trust I do not propose to touch, but I wish to say a very few words of the hopes and wishes of scientific men and physicians with regard to it. From the time of the first announcement of the Hopkins bequests to the present, these men, all over the world, have been keenly interested in the plans and methods adopted in carrying them out. Whenever and wherever the problems of higher medical education have been discussed within the last ten years, there has been speculation as to the probable course of the Johns Hopkins medical department, and the influence it would have upon the standard. I may even say that some of this influence has been exerted in advance—has been discounted, as it were—for the plans of this Hospital have stimulated changes in some of our best medical schools, and have been copied with more or less modification in some of our latest hospitals.

What is it, then, that the physicians want? They hope that the Hopkins Medical School and Hospital will do two things. The first is, that it will demand of those who propose to become its students evidence that they have a sound basis of preliminary education before they commence, and that its standard in this respect shall be little below that of the requirements for granting the degree of bachelor of arts in the University. It is hoped that the men thus selected will go through a carefully graded course of study, including actual work in properly fitted laboratories, and that after this they will be brought into contact with the sick, and thus obtain practical experience of the duties and responsibilities of the practitioner of medicine before they offer their services as such to the public.

So much our physicians desire of every medical

school, for the sake of the honor and dignity of the profession, and for the good of the public, and they desire especially that this school shall form an example to which they can point as showing how medical education should be conducted, and what should be required of the candidate for the degree of doctor of medicine.

The very general interest in the combined Hopkins trusts felt by the physicians and scientific men not only of this country, but of the whole civilized world, is largely due to the belief that the relations which will here exist and be maintained between the University as a whole and its medical department, of which this Hospital is to be an important part, will be close and intimate, so that the true university spirit will pervade, stimulate and encourage the hospital work. In this country medical schools have either had no connection with universities properly so-called, or the connection has been slight and nominal, such as depends upon the formal conferring of medical degrees by the university. Here, however, through the influence of the biological department, there are secured common interests and mutual influence, and it is hoped, therefore, that the necessary details of technological instruction will be arranged in accordance with and subordinate to the broad principles of scientific culture upon which this University is organized.

It is because it is believed that this will be the case that there is a widespread hope and expectation that these combined institutions will endeavor to produce investigators as well as practitioners, to give the world men who can not only sail by the old charts, but who can make new and better ones for the use of others. This can only be done where the professors and teachers are themselves seeking to increase knowledge, and doing this for the sake of the knowledge itself;—and hence it is supposed that from this Hospital will issue papers and reports giving accounts of advances in, and new methods of acquiring knowledge, obtained in its wards and laboratories, and that thus all scientific men and all physicians shall share in the benefits of the work actually done within these walls. But, however interesting and valuable this work may be in itself, it is of secondary importance to the future of science and medicine and to the world at large, in comparison with the production of trained investigators, full of enthusiasm, and imbued with the spirit of scientific research, who will spread the influence of such training far and wide. It is to young men thus fitted for the work that we look for the solution of some of the myriad problems which now confront the biologist and the physician.

Do I seem to ask too much? to be too sanguine as to what human thought and study, and skill may accomplish? to forget that there is one event unto all; that the shadow of pain and death comes on the wise man as on the fool? I have two answers. As surely as our improved methods of prevention and treatment, based on the advances in knowledge of the last fifty years, have already extended the average duration of life in civilized countries nearly five years, have prolonged thousands of useful and productive lives, and have done away with the indescribable agonies of the pre-anaesthetic period, so surely we are on the verge of still greater advances, especially in the prevention of infectious and contagious disease, in the resources of surgery against deformities and morbid growths, and in the mitigation of suffering due to causes which cannot be wholly removed. But the second answer is more important, and it is this: It is our duty to try to increase and diffuse knowledge according to the means and opportunities which we have, and not to rest idle because we cannot certainly foresee that we shall reap where we have strewn. "It is not incumbent on thee to finish the work, but thou must not therefore depart from it," says the Talmud, and "Of him to whom much is given much shall be required," says the Scripture.

To you, the officers of this institution, and to you, men and women of Baltimore, there is now given the opportunity of giving powerful aid in this increase and diffusion of knowledge of the laws of human life, disease and death. Surely, those who are working in the wards and laboratories of the Hospital and University will do their best; surely, also, the citizens of this great city, of a great nation, which at no distant day will take the lead in scientific work, will encourage, sustain and sympathize with these workers. I would have this Hospital become famous, not for fame's sake, but because this will be evidence of the good work which has been done in it; but we must not be impatient. There are difficulties to be overcome, delays which must be submitted to. We cannot at once have the Medical School which is essential to the plan which I have sketched; but there is plenty to do for the present, and I am certain that in time all these present obstacles to full development will be happily overcome.

Success in this, as in all other enterprises in this world, is to be obtained by unselfish work for the good of others, by wise counsel, by cooperation, and by persistent effort.

A hospital is a living organism, made up of many different parts having different functions, but all these must be in due proportion and relation to each other, and to the environment, to produce the desired general results. The stream of life which runs through it is incessantly changing; patients and nurses and doctors come and go; to-day it has to deal with the results of an epidemic, tomorrow with those of an explosion or fire; the reputation of its physicians or surgeons attracts those suffering from a peculiar form of disease, and as the one changes so do others. Its work is never done; its equipment is never complete; it is always in need of new means of diagnosis, of new instruments and medicines; it is to try all things and hold fast to that which is good.

It has been said that "hospitals are in some sort the measure of the civilization of a people," but a hospital of this kind should be more than an index. It should be an active force in the community in which it is placed. When the mediaeval priest established in each great city in France a Hotel Dieu, a place for God's hospitality, it was in the interests of charity as he understood it, including both the helping of the sick poor and the affording to those who were neither sick nor poor an opportunity and a stimulus to help their fellow men; and doubtless the cause of humanity and religion was advanced more by the effect on the givers than on the receivers. It is the old lesson so often expounded, apparently so simple and yet so hard to learn, that true happiness lies in helping others; that it is more blessed to give than to receive.

In some respects we to-day have a much wider outlook than the men of a thousand years ago. This Hospital is designed, as I have told you, to advance medical science as well as to give relief to the sick poor, but the fundamental motive is the same—to help others.

We have here the beginning of an institution which shall endure long after the speakers and the audience of to-day shall have finished their life-work and have passed away. Founded in the interest of suffering humanity, intimately connected with a great University, amply provided with what is at present known to be essential to its work, we have every reason to predict for it a long and prosperous career, with steadily progressing improvement in its organization and methods, and enlargement of its activity and influence.

Let us hope that before the last sands have run out from beneath the feet of the years of the nineteenth century it will have become a model of its kind, and that upon the centennial of its anniversary it will be a hospital which shall still compare favorably, not only in structure and arrangement, but also in results achieved, with any other institution of like character in existence. (*Applause.*)

(*As the applause ceases, Mr. King rises and steps forward.*)

*Mr. King:* The next and last speaker of this morning's exercises needs no introduction to this audience. During the fourteen years that he has been a resident of this city he has by his accomplishments and his character earned the respect and admiration of all right-thinking citizens of this community. Within the short space of scarcely a decade and a half he has organized and set in operation a new university which has already won for itself a unique place in American institutions of higher learning. He has shown such great ability in the field of educational administration that it was but natural that the Board of Trustees of the Hospital should turn to him to oganize the administrative service of that institution. He graciously consented to give of his time and energy for this work, and the Trustees of the University, at the request of the Trustees of the Hospital, kindly released him for a time for this service. Since January of this year he has devoted himself to the task, an altogether unique undertaking for a University president, I should judge, and I think I may say that the contribution which he has made to this Hospital in the organization of its essential administrative services, and in the selection of the men who are to serve as the heads of its professional services, will rank as second only to his great services to its sister institution, the University. It gives me great pleasure to present to you Dr. Daniel C. Gilman, President of the Johns Hopkins University. (*Applause.*)

*Mr. Gilman:* (*advances with manuscript in his hand and reads*) Ladies and Gentlemen: Thirteen years ago during the centennial celebrations of Independence Day, the University founded by Johns Hopkins began its work, and now, as we commemorate a completed century of constitutional life, the Hospital, gift of the same donor, throws open its doors. These buildings,—on which thought, time and wealth have been freely spent—are now consecrated to the ministry of mercy and the prolongation of life. Science and charity, knowledge and pity, skill and sympathy are here installed in the service of mankind.

That large-minded citizen of Maryland, "who by noble gifts for the advancement of learning and the relief of suffering, has won the gratitude of his city and his country," found two words adequate to his great ideas. "University" and

"Hospital" were his chosen terms, and he linked them together by this significant phrase: "Bear constantly in mind that it is my wish and purpose that the hospital shall ultimately form a part of the medical school of the university for which I have made ample provision by my will." How brief the phrase, how large the purpose! "Apples of gold in pictures of silver."

Like James Henry Roosevelt of New York, "a man upright in his aims, simple in his life and sublime in his benefactions," whose hospital and dispensary give clinical instruction to the College of Physicians and Surgeons; like James Lenox of New York, whose munificence established a public library and gave birth to a hospital, Johns Hopkins, already honored as a patron of learning, will be henceforward remembered in the annals of charity and medicine. May we not almost say of him as Pindar said of Theron,

—and I will swear
That city none,—tho' she unroll,
A century past, her radiant scroll,—
Hath brought a mortal man to light
Whose hand with larger bounty flows.
The blessings to that man we owe
Say who shall hope to count.

We may form an idea of what this hospital may become by the study of a like institution in London. About a century and a half before Johns Hopkins died, the days of Thomas Guy were ended. Like our benefactor, he had lived unmarried to the age of eighty years, and from humble beginnings had acquired a fortune, with which he provided for the establishment of a hospital. The amount of his gift was more than a million of dollars (238,292 pounds). The beneficent influence of Guy's hospital is now known in every part of the globe. It is doubtless safe to say that every one of us has shared, indirectly, in its benefits. The name of the great surgeon, Sir Astley Cooper, would alone give renown to the hospital to which he was attached,—Sir Astley Cooper, of whom it was said that from the period of his appointment to Guy's until the moment of his latest breath, he was everything and all to the suffering and afflicted; his name was a host; but his presence brought confidence and comfort. Addison and Hodgkins, whose names are familiar to the historians of medicine, were physicians in that hospital. So was Richard Bright whose discoveries have been pronounced the most important contribution to medical science, made in the first half of the nineteenth century. The observations and studies made in Guy's Hospital since 1836 fill fifty volumes. Thousands of medical students have been trained within its walls. "Their presence," says a competent observer, "has made the hospital." Hundreds of thousands of patients have received relief from the treatment there afforded. In a single year, five thousand indoor patients have been cared for and more than thirty thousand outdoor patients have sought advice.

But we are planning for a future much longer than a century and a half; for a history as long as that of St. Bartholomew's or St. Thomas's, which now, after many centuries, are more useful than ever.

By a curious coincidence, as I had reached this point in the preparation of my address, I received a volume from Dr. Norman Moore, the Warden of St. Bartholomew's Hospital in London—bearing an inscription so welcome and so apposite that I will read it. "To the library of the newest of Hospitals this account of the progress of medicine in one of the most ancient is given by Norman Moore, with the earnest hope that the Johns Hopkins Hospital may flourish at least as long as the Royal Hospital of St. Bartholomew, in Smithfield, and prove no less useful to mankind,—on the opening day of the Johns Hopkins Hospital, 1889."

Time may efface the personality of our founder,

as it has effaced the personality of Rahere, the founder of St. Bartholomew's, but the beneficence of Johns Hopkins will last for centuries; and gratitude will cherish the memory of his broad views, his great liberality, his wise and beneficent purposes.

The previous speakers have told us of the circumstances which led to the construction of these buildings and have described their purposes. Let me from a different point of view point out some of the benefits which are likely to proceed from this foundation.

First, last and always, this Hospital is to furnish relief to the sick and wounded. Make the best of it, introduce fresh air and sunshine, and provide the utmost comfort, secure wise physicians, engage the best trained nurses, decorate the walls with pictures, bring fruit and flowers and books and friends,—and even the comforting influence of Religion, yet you cannot conceal the direful consciousness, that this is the house of suffering.

From any other ill,
(Except it be remorse) can man escape
By work,—the healing of divinest balm
To whom so hath the courage to begin:—
But sickness holds the sick man in a chain
No will can break or bend to earthly use.

The names that have been given to these abodes of the sick are suggestive. Hospitality and hospital alike suggest the bestowal of kindness to guests. The word Lazaretto, ultimately degraded, pointed at first to the restoration of life. Misericordia, la Charité, la Pitié, the Home of the Good Samaritan, the House of Mercy, bring to mind the kindly influences of love and care.

By whatever name it may be called this is a convent where sickness is the abbess. The rule of sympathy for the suffering must govern everybody with a strictness of discipline as rigid as the rule of the Benedictines or the Carthusians. Those who daily walk these cloisters will be the warders of life and health, however high their station or however humble their service; and casual visitors will not cross the threshold of the wards without pity for those who are disabled or without admiration and gratitude for those whose lives are spent in alleviating distress.

This Hospital will not only meet the daily calls of humanity, it will stand ready to render extraordinary services in those emergencies which not even the progress of municipal reform and preventive medicine can entirely ward off. A fire, an explosion, an accident on the rails or on the seashore, the fall of a platform or of a building poorly constructed, may at any moment tax the utmost resources of a great establishment. True, we have no fear of leprosy and the plague; we have almost ceased to dread the coming of cholera; yellow fever, we are hoping to thwart in its approaches to our northern seaports;—vaccination, which was spoken of by Sir James Simpson, "as the greatest thought ever broached in practical medicine," is a great prophylactic; but we are not certain that diphtheria and infectious fevers will not continue to be epidemic; nor can we always be sure that the boards of health in the city and State, will succeed in protecting us, as well as they can, from the inroads of pestilence. Indeed it is well to inquire whether Baltimore is now fortified as it should be against the hostile incursions of epidemic disease. In addition to its other functions, this Hospital will stand as a reserved force, a sort of storehouse of energy, ready to serve the city if apprehension and disease spread their pall upon it.

This Hospital would be a very narrow institution if it kept to itself its experience. It is the essence of quackery to deal in mysteries and nostrums; it is the glory of medicine that it owns no patents and conceals no discoveries. On the contrary, the best hospitals of the world consider it one of their first duties — second only to the care of their patients — to record the cases they have treated, the methods they have pursued, the results whether favorable or unfavorable which have followed. Scientific studies in pathology and practical medicine must be printed. Special papers, often requiring costly illustrations, must be published upon extraordinary cases, and upon new operations and modes of relief. It is thus that the science of Medicine is advanced. Where secrecy reigns, carelessness and ignorance delight to hide; skill loves the light.

It is impossible to have a hospital without its becoming a place for medical education. It is interesting to note that in the physician's oath, attributed to Hippocrates, the duty of imparting knowledge is explicitly enforced. Even the country doctor as he rides from village to village, takes in his gig an observing pupil, like the squire to a knight-errant. Every great surgeon is watched with the closest attention by the younger physicians who assist him. Every mother is the pupil of the physician whom she calls upon to attend her suffering child. So, of course, a hospital, having upon its staff men of rare qualifications who are in daily consultation with their most skilful brethren, is, from the necessities of the case, a place for instruction. How systematic that instruction will be depends on circumstances that at the moment need not be presented. All that need now be said is that hospitals the wide world over are the schools of medicine and surgery.

The training of nurses is another form of hospital activity, recently developed, never hence to be abandoned. To the sisterhoods of the Roman Catholic Church, to the Protestant Deaconesses of Kaiserswerth and the Bethanien at Berlin, and to many guilds in many lands, much credit is due for lessons they have taught the world, as to the importance of training nurses. Elizabeth Fry was one of the first Englishwomen to propose such instruc- struction. Florence Nightingale, by her services in the Crimean War, and by her subsequent writings, has borne a noble part in this work. So, too, have our own countrywomen. The Civil War, full of sad recollections, has some bright stories, and among them none more inspiring than the labors of brave, self-sacrificing and intelligent women in the hospitals. Who that has read "What we did at Gettysburg," or "Hospital Days," has forgotten their lessons? As a direct result of the war, Nurses' Schools have grown up in every part of this land. Our Hospital has such a department soon to be opened, where nurses will be trained, not only for their merciful offices within these walls but for household engagements and for visiting among the poor.

A good hospital may readily become the rallying place of the medical profession who are resident in the city.

"Through mutual intercourse and mutual aid
Great deeds are done and great discoveries made;
The wise new wisdom on the wise bestow
Whilst the lone thinker's thoughts come slight
and slow."

One purpose of this central building is to afford opportunities for professional intercourse. Here are rooms set apart for the library that will presently be collected; here the medical journals will be taken in; here are the best appliances and instruments for the treatment of patients; here are rooms for private consultations and for public conferences; here are laboratories for physiological and pathological determinations; and it will not surprise me to hear that within a very short time medical associations are here brought together "for mutual intercourse and mutual aid" at the invitation of Dr. Osler, the physician in chief, who this day assumes his great responsibility with the hearty welcome of Baltimoreans, and with the well-earned confidence of the profession throughout the entire land.

From the past let us turn to the future. All the signs of the times point to a new era in the history of mankind. All the sciences are leading up to a better understanding of the laws of life, to a true Anthropology, and the consequent improvement of the physical, mental and moral powers of man.

There are four or five directions toward which we may turn an expectant gaze, as in days gone by the merchants watched upon the house tops for the return of the ships they had sent out to distant ports.

Preventive medicine promises to do more and more for mankind. As the germs of many specific disorders have been discovered, so the means of their destruction have been found out. If legislature and civil administration keep up with science, if knowledge is controlled by virtue and followed by temperance, the community will be freed from many of the foes which in former generations have slain their tens of thousands.

From the chemical laboratory new remedies, as well as simpler forms of old remedies, are to be constantly looked for. The synthetical processes which now receive so much attention have lately made important contributions to the pharmacopeia. It would surprise any one whose attention has not been directed to this point to know how many claimants are awaiting judgment. Scores of substances, till lately unknown, as I have heard my colleague, Professor Remsen, say, are awaiting the study of competent therapeutists. Nobody can foretell what will come from their new contributions to materia medica, but one who watches the processes of discovery must feel certain that secrets hid from the beginning are ere long to be revealed, and that many of the substances already discovered have properties of the most serviceable character.

No one can say what will result from the attention that has been recently given to the study of physical phenomena by the exact methods of science,—but the outlook is hopeful. If we are as far as ever from elucidating the mysterious interrelationship of the mind and the body, progress has certainly been made in a knowledge of the laws by which they act upon each other. The knowledge that has been acquired in respect to the functions of the brain and nervous system has already led to the treatment of many disorders and the relief of many diseases which a short time ago were beyond the reach of remedy. We are not without hope that in the physiological and psychophysical laboratories already established here, important contributions will be made to science which will ultimately prove to be of value to medicine and to the conduct of the body in health and disease.

In the near future we are to look for progress in the applications of electricity and magnetism to the treatment of disease as well as to its diagnosis. Chemistry by its synthetic methods is producing new remedies, which experimental therapeutics proceeds to test, and pharmacy then appropriates. The laws of light, heat, electricity and magnetism are found in close relationship to the problems of relief and cure. The laws of temperature and climate have their services to render. Even the influence of barometrical pressure upon surgical operations begins to be noticed. The study of the nervous system is sure at no distant day, to make important contributions to the welfare of man. Psychology is waiting for the results. Experimental physiology is doing its part. Pathology, a term as old as Hippocrates, has become a new science within the last few years. The laws of descent have but just begun to assume a scientific form. Preventive medicine is almost a new conception. The morality of personal hygiene is a new department of ethics. Biology, after having met with the same critical reception with which anatomy, astronomy, geology and chronology were greeted, may yet be honored as leading to the highest and noblest conceptions of humanity; anthropology, and the knowledge of man in his relations to the universe in which he is placed, may sum up finite knowledge.

So all along the line, in the laboratories of the university and in the wards of the hospital, knowledge is contributing to the welfare of man. The days of the coming man may not always reach the full allotment to which Chevreul has just attained, but perhaps to die at seventy will be to die in youth, and to reach the age of eighty or ninety in health and vigor, will be the rule and not the exception. Nor is length of days our only hope. The disappearance of epidemics, fewer days of confinement in sickness, fewer "minor ailments," a decrease of infantile mortality, greater powers of resistance to the evils of certain occupations, and comparative immunity from many infirmities which are now common, artificial reinforcements and replacements of bodily defects, simpler and surer means of diagnosis, the detection of the nature, origin and history of specific affections,—and finally the assurance of euthanasia. These, as it seems to a layman, are reasonable expectations which the nineteenth century holds out to the twentieth. Can any outlay be too great if humanity is thus benefited?

To the attainment of these noble aims, "the relief of suffering and the advancement of knowledge," the foundations of Johns Hopkins are forever set apart. On the one hand stands the University, where education in the liberal arts and sciences is provided, and where research is liberally encouraged; on the other hand stands the Hospital, where all that art and science can contribute to the relief of sickness and pain is bountifully provided. Is there anything wanting? Yes,—there is still a great want to be supplied, an arch to rest upon these pillars. An Institute of Medicine and Surgery, a College of Physicians and Surgeons, a Medical School,—the office of which shall be to promote the training of young physicians, and the encouragement of medical science is imperatively needed. Is it too much to say that there is not such an opportunity on the globe, for another Peabody or another Hopkins to benefit his fellow man?

The University needs all it has, and more, to carry on the non-professional courses to which its funds are appropriated. The hospital, with all its readiness to cooperate in the advancement of knowledge, will, after all, remain as I have said before, and cannot say with too much emphasis,—the home of the sick, the feeble, the injured and the dying. It is the house of mercy, not the hall of philosophy. But in close alliance with both these foundations there is a place for a School of Medicine, which may bear its founder's name, and may render services as significant and memorable as those of Salerno and Bologna, at the beginning of the modern era; as those of Leyden and Edinburgh where the earliest American physicians received their education; or as those of Berlin and Vienna to which so many students of this decade resort.

This grateful city should no longer delay placing upon one of the squares near the monument of Washington, the figure of Johns Hopkins, with such designs as an artist, and an artist only, could devise, to typify the great ideas which underlie his gifts,—"the advancement of knowledge and the relief of suffering." Then might some friend of this Hospital place beneath this dome a copy of Thorwaldsen's Christus Consolator, with the outstretched hands of mercy, to remind each passer-by —the physician and the nurse as they pursue their ministry of relief; the student as he begins his daily task; and the sufferer from injury or disease, that over all this institution rests the perpetual benediction of Christian charity, the constant spirit of "good will to man." Upon one hill of Baltimore rises a temple, "Whose guardian crest, the silent cross," is an emblem of the Christian faith; upon another, a lofty column reminds us of the patriots' hope; upon a third, the Hotel-Dieu is placed,—the house of charity. Significant triad! "Here abideth Faith, Hope and Charity, but the greatest of these is Charity." (*Applause.*)

*Mr. King:* (*rises and comes forward*) I shall now call upon His Excellency, the Governor of Maryland, to open the Hospital officially. Ladies and Gentlemen, the Honorable Elihu E. Jackson, Governor of Maryland. (*Returns to his seat as the company applauds.*)

*Governor Jackson:* (*rises and comes forward*) Ladies and Gentlemen: By act of the General Assembly of the State of Maryland, passed in January, 1867, authority was granted for the formation of a corporation known as The Johns Hopkins Hospital. That Hospital has now come into being and I hereby declare it open and dedicated to the service of humanity. May it never close! And I congratulate the citizens of Baltimore upon now having the newest and the finest hospital in the world! (*Bows. Applause.*)

CURTAIN.